The Vibrant KETO Chaffle Cooking Guide

Keto-friendly Chaffle Recipes For Weight Loss

Lily Sherman

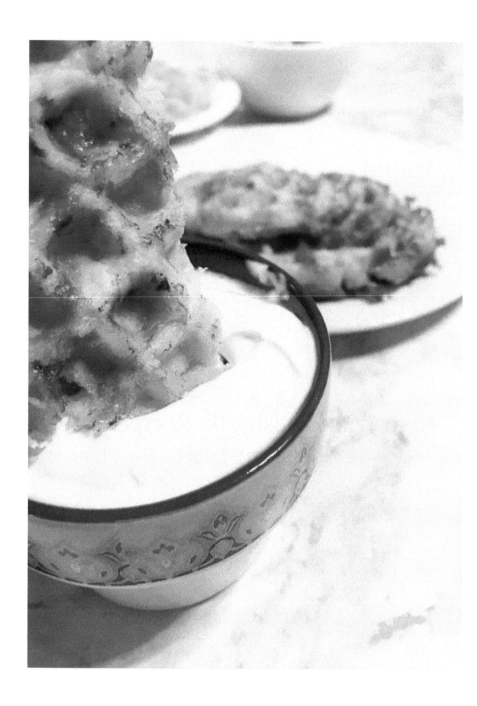

Table of contents

Buffalo Chicken Chaffles 7

Garlic And Spinach chaffles 9

Chaffle Sandwich 11

Cauliflower & Italian Seasoning..13

Chaffle Cuban Sandwich 15

Protein Chaffles 17

Tuna Chaffles 19

Sausage & Veggie Chaffles..21

Bit Chaffle Sandwich 23

Keto Pepperoni Pizza Chaffle... 26

Easy Chaffle with Keto Sausage Gravy 28

BLT Keto Chaffle Sandwich 31

Mini Keto Pizza 33

Aioli Chicken Chaffle Sandwich 35

Sage & Coconut Milk Chaffles...37

Chaffle Burger... 39

Best Keto Pizza Chaffle... 42

Keto Taco Chaffle with Crispy Taco Shells 45

Chaffle Keto Protein Chaffle...47

Garlic Mayo Vegan Chaffles 49

Best Vegan Keto Chaffle 51

Cauliflower Chaffles & Tomatoes... 53

Broccoli & Cheese Chaffles 55

Scallion - Coconut Chaffles 57

Asian Cauliflower Chaffles 59

Mushroom and Almond Chaffle 61

Spinach and Artichoke Chaffle 63

Jicama Vegetarian Keto Chaffle 65

Jicama Loaded Baked Potato Chaffle 67

Lettuce Chaffles Sandwich 69

Vegan Chaffles With Flaxseed 71

Crispy Bagel Chaffles 73

Garlic and Onion Powder Chaffles 75

Savory Bagel Seasoning Chaffles 77

Dried Herbs Chaffle 79

Zucchini & Basil Chaffles 81

Hash Brown Chaffle 83

Almonds and Flaxseeds Chaffles 85

Broccoli Chaffle 87

Garlic Bread Chaffle 89

Cinnamon Chaffle Rolls 92

Broccoli & Almond Flour Chaffles 94

Cheddar Jalapeño Chaffle 96

Rosemary in Chaffles 98

Zucchini in Chaffles 100

Avocado Croque Madam Chaffle 102

5

Fruity Vegan Chaffles 104

Vegan Chocolate Chaffles 106

Apple Cinnamon Chaffles.. 108

Blueberry Chaffles 110

Buffalo Chicken Chaffles

Cooking: 5 Minutes

Servings: 4

Ingredients

- 1/4 cup almond flour
- 1 tsp baking powder
- 2 large eggs
- 1/2 cup chicken, shredded
- 1/4 cup sharp cheddar cheese, shredded
- 1/4 cup mozzarella cheese, shredded
- 1/4 cup Red-Hot Sauce " 1 Tbsp for TOPPING
- 1/4 cup feta cheese, crumbled
- 1/4 cup celery, diced

Directions

1. Whisk baking powder and almond flour in a tiny bowl and set aside.
2. Turn on waffle maker to heat and oil it with cooking spray.
3. Beat eggs in a large bowl until frothy.

4. Add hot sauce and beat until combined.

5. Mix in flour mixture.

6. Add cheeses and Mix well until well combined.

7. Fold in chicken.

8. Pour batter into waffle maker and cook for 4 minutes.

9. Remove now and repeat until all batter is used up.

10. Top with celery, feta, and hot sauce.

Nutrition:

Calories: 337, Carbs: 4 g, Fat: 2 6 g, Protein: 22 g,

Garlic And Spinach chaffles

Cooking: 5 minutes

Servings: 2

Ingredients

- 1 cup egg whites.
- 1 tsp Italian spice
- 2 tsps. coconut flour
- 1/2 tsp vanilla
- 1 tsp baking powder
- 1 tsp baking soda
- 1 cup mozzarella cheese, grated
- 1/2 tsp garlic powder
- 1 cup chopped spinach

Directions

1. Switch on your square waffle maker. Spray with non-stick spray.
2. Beat egg whites with beater, until fluffy and white.
3. Add pumpkin puree, pumpkin pie spice, coconut flour in egg whites and beat again.

4. Stir in the cheese, powder, garlic powder, baking soda, and powder.
5. Sprinkle chopped spinach on a warm maker
6. Pour the batter in waffle maker over chopped spinach
7. Close the maker and cook for about 4-5 minutes.
8. Remove now chaffles from the maker.
9. Serve hot and enjoy!

Nutrition:

Protein: 52 % 88kcal, Fat: 41% 69 kcal, Carbohydrates: 7% 12 kcal

Chaffle Sandwich

Cooking: 8 Minutes

Servings: 2

Ingredients

Chaffle bread:

- 1/2 cup mozzarella cheese, shredded
- 1 egg
- 1 tbs green onion, diced
- 1/2 tsp Italian seasoning

Sandwich:

- 1/2 lb bacon, pre-cooked
- 1 tiny lettuce
- 1 medium tomato sliced
- 1 tbsp mayo

Directions

1. Preheat now your mini waffle maker
2. Whip the egg in a tiny mixing bowl
3. Add the seasonings, cheese, and onion. Mix thoroughly until it's well incorporated

4. Add a teaspn of shredded cheese to your waffle maker and cook for 30 seconds
5. Place half the batter in the waffle pan and cook for 4 minutes
6. Once the first chaffle is done, repeat the process with the chaffle
7. Once ready Remove now and place on a plate. Top with the mayo, lettuce, bacon, and tomato.
8. Place the second chaffle on top, slice into 2 and enjoy!

Nutrition:

Calories: 240Kcal, Fats: 18 g, Carbs: 2 g, Protein: 17 g

Cauliflower & Italian Seasoning

Cooking: 20 Minutes

Servings: 4

Ingredients

- 1 cup cauliflower rice
- 1/4 teaspn garlic powder
- 1/2 teaspn Italian seasoning
- Salt and freshy ground black pepper to taste
- 1/2 cup Parmesan cheese, shredded

Directions

1. Preheat now a mini waffle iron and details, you fit money
2. In a blender, add the Ingredients except parmesan cheese and pulse until well combined
3. Place 1.1/2 tbspn of the Parmesan
4. Put Cheese in the bottom of Preheat nowed waffle iron.
5. Place 1/4 of the egg mixture over cheese and sprinkle with the 1/2 tbspn of the Parmesan cheese.
6. Cook for about 4-minutes or until golden brown.

7. Repeat now with the remaining mixture and Parmesan cheese.
8. Serve warm.

Nutrition:

Calories: 127, Net Carb: 2g, Fat: 9g, Saturated Fat: 5.3g, Carbohydrates: 2.7g, Dietary Fiber: 0.7g, Sugar: 1.5g, Protein: 9.2g

Chaffle Cuban Sandwich

Cooking: 10 minutes

Servings: 1

Ingredients

- 1 Large egg
- 1 Tbsp almond flour
- 1 Tbsp Full-fat greek yogurt
- 1/4 tsp baking powder
- 1/4 cup shredded swiss cheese

For the filling:

- 3 oz roast pork
- 2 oz deli ham
- 1 slice swiss chance
- 3-5 sliced pickle hip
- 3 oz roast pork
- 2 oz deli ham
- 1 slice Swiss cheese
- 3-5 sliced pickle chips
- 1/2 Tbsp Dijon mustard

Directions

1. Turn on waffle maker to heat and oil it with cooking spray.
2. Beat egg, yogurt, almond flour, and baking powder in a bowl.
3. Sprinkle 1/4 swiss cheese on hot waffle maker. Top with half of the egg mixture, then add 4 of the cheese on top. Close and cook for 5 min, until brown and crispy.
4. Repeat now with remaining batter.
5. Layer pork, ham, and cheese slice in a tiny microwaveable bowl. Microwave for seconds, until cheese Mels.
6. Spread the inside of chaffle with mustard and top with pickles. Invert bowl onto Chaffle top so that cheese is touching pickles. Place bottom chaffle onto pork and serve.

Nutrition:

Carbs: 4 g, Fat: 46 g, Protein: 33g, Calories: 522

Protein Chaffles

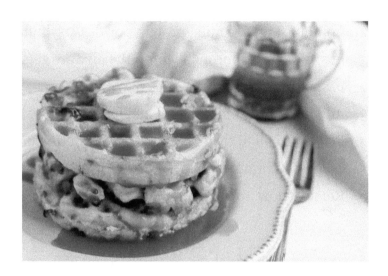

Cooking: 4 Minutes

Servings: 1

Ingredients

- 1/4 cup almond milk
- 1/4 cup plant-based protein powder
- 2 tbsp almond butter
- 1 tbsp psyllium husk

Directions

1. Preheat now your waffle maker.
2. Combine almond milk, protein powder, psyllium husk, and mix thoroughly until the mixture gets a paste form.
3. Add in butter, combine well and form round balls
4. Place the ball in the center of Preheat waffle maker.
5. Cook for 4 minutes.
6. Remove now, top as prefer and enjoy.

Nutrition:

Calories: 310 Kcal, Fats: 19 g, Carbs: 5 g, Protein: 25 g

Tuna Chaffles

Cooking: 9 Minutes

Servings: 2

Ingredients

- 1 organic egg, beaten
- 1/2 cup plus 2 teaspns Mozzarella cheese, shredded and divided
- 1 (2.6-ounce of) can water-packed tuna, drained
- Pinch of salt

Directions

1. Preheat now a mini waffle iron and then grease it.
2. In a bowl, place the egg, 1/2 cup of mozzarella cheese, tuna and salt and mix well
3. Place 1 teaspn of Mozzarella cheese in the bottom of Preheat nowed waffle iron and cook for about seconds.
4. Place the egg mixture over cheese and cook for about minutes or until golden brown.
5. Repeat now with the remaining mixture.
6. Serve warm.

Nutrition:

Calories: 94, Net Carb: 0.4g, Fat: 3g, Saturated Fat: 1.5g, Carbohydrates: 0.4g, Dietary Fiber: 0g, Sugar: 0.2g, Protein: 14.2g

Sausage & Veggie Chaffles

Cooking: 20 Minutes

Servings: 4

Ingredients

- 1/3 cup of unsweetened almond milk.
- 4 medium organic eggs
- 2 tbsps gluten-free breakfast.
- sausage, cut into slices
- 2 tbsps broccoli florets, chopped
- 2 tbsps bell peppers, seeded and chopped
- 2 tbsps mozzarella cheese, shredded

Directions

1. Preheat now a waffle iron and then grease it.
2. In a bowl, add the almond milk, eggs and beat well.
3. Place the remaining Ingredients and stir to combine well.
4. Place desired amount of the mixture into Preheat waffle iron.
5. Cook for about minutes.

6. Repeat now with the remaining batter

7. Serve warm.

Nutrition:

Calories 132, Net Carbs 1.2 g, Total Fat 9.2 g, Saturated Fat 3.5 g, Sodium 216 mg, Total Carbs 1.4 g, Fiber 0.2 g, Sugar 0.5 g, Protein 11.1 g

Bit Chaffle Sandwich

Cooking: 10 Minutes

Servings: 1

Ingredients

Sandwich Filling:

- 2 strips of bacon
- A pinch of salt
- 2 slices tomato
- 1 tbsp mayonnaise
- 3 pieces lettuce

Chaffle:

- 1 egg (beaten)
- 1/2 cup shredded mozzarella cheese
- 1/4 tsp onion powder
- 1/4 tsp garlic powder
- 1/2 tsp curry powder

Directions:

1. Plug your waffle maker and Preheat now it. Spray it with a non-stick spray.

2. In a mixing bowl, combine the cheese, onion powder, garlic and curry powder. Add the egg and mix well until the Ingredients are well combined.

3. Fill your waffle maker with the batter and spread the batter to your waffle maker's edges to cover all the holes on the waffle iron.

4. Close your waffle maker's lid and cook for about minutes or according to waffle maker's settings.

5. After the cooking cycle, remove now the chaffle from your waffle maker using a silicone or plastic utensil.

6. Repeat step 3 to 5 until you have cooked all the batter into chaffles. Set the chaffles aside to cool.

7. Heat up a skillet over medium heat. Add the bacon strips and sear until all bacon sides are browned, turning and pressing the bacon while searing.

8. Use a slotted spoon to transfer the bacon to a paper towel lined plate to drain.

9. Place the chaffles on a flat surface and spread mayonnaise over the face of the chaffles.

10. Divide the lettuce into two and layer it on one portion on both chaffles.

11. Layer the tomatoes on one of the chaffles and sprinkle with salt. Layer the bacon over the tomatoes and place the other chaffle over the one containing the bacon.

12. Press and serve immediately.

13. Enjoy!!!

Nutrition:

Carbohydrate 7.8g 3%, Sugars 2.7g, Protein 18.4g

Keto Pepperoni Pizza Chaffle

Preparation: 10 minutes

Servings: 2

Ingredients

- 1 egg
- 1/2 cup mozzarella cheese shredded
- Just a pinch of Italian seasoning
- No sugar added pizza sauce about 1 tbspn
- Top with more shredded cheese pepperoni

Directions

1. Preheat now the waffle maker.
2. In a tiny bowl, whip the egg and seasonings together.
3. Mix in the shredded cheese.
4. Add a tsp of shredded cheese to the Preheat waffle maker and let it cook for about 30 seconds. This will help to create a crisper crust.
5. Add half the mixture to your waffle maker and cook it for about 4 minutes until it's golden brown and slightly crispy!

6. Remove now the waffle and add the remaining mixture to your waffle maker to make the second chaffle.
7. Top with a tbspn of pizza sauce, shredded cheese, and pepperoni. Microwave it on high for about 20 seconds.

Nutrition:

Calories: 76 kcal, Carbohydrates: 4.1g, Protein: 5.5g, Fat: 4.3g, Fiber: 1.2g, Sugar: 1.9g

Easy Chaffle with Keto Sausage Gravy

Preparation: 5 minutes

Cooking: 10 minutes

Ingredients

For the Chaffle:

- 1 egg
- 1/2 cup mozzarella cheese, grated
- 1 tsp coconut flour
- 1 tsp water
- 1/4 tsp baking powder
- pinch of salt

For the Keto Sausage Gravy:

- 1/4 cup breakfast sausage, browned
- 3 tbsp chicken broth
- 2 tbsp heavy whipping cream
- 2 tsp cream cheese, softened
- dash garlic powder
- pepper to taste
- dash of onion powder (optional)

Directions

1. Plug Waffle Maker into the wall and allow to heat up. Grease lightly or use cooking spray.

2. Combine all the Ingredients for the chaffle into a tiny bowl and stir to combine well.

3. Pour half of the chaffle batter onto your waffle maker, then shut the lid and cook for approx 4 minutes.

4. Remove now chaffle from waffle maker and repeat the same process to make the second chaffle. Set aside to crisp.

5. For the Keto Sausage Gravy

6. Cook one pound of breakfast sausage and drain. Reserve 1/4 cup for this .

7. Make sausage patties out of the rest of the sausage and reserve 1/4 a cup to brown for this. If you aren't familiar with breakfast sausage, it is crumbled like ground beef.

8. Wipe excess grease from the skillet and add 1/4 cup browned breakfast sausage and the rest of the Ingredients and bring to a boil stirring continuously.

9. Reduce heat to medium and continue to cook down with the lid off so that it begins to thicken for approximately 5-7 minutes. If you'd like it very thick, you can add a bit of Xanthan Gum, but if you are

patient with it simmering the keto sausage gravy will thicken. Then, it will thicken even more as it cools.

10. Add salt and pepper to taste and spoon keto sausage gravy over chaffles.

11. Enjoy

Nutrition:

Calories: 212 kcal, Carbohydrates: 3g, Protein: 11g, Fat: 17g, Saturated Fat: 10g, Cholesterol: 134mg, Sodium: 350mg, Potassium: 133mg, Fiber: 1g, Sugar: 1g, Vitamin A: 595IU, Vitamin C: 2mg, Calcium: 191mg, Iron: 1mg

BLT Keto Chaffle Sandwich

Preparation: 3 minutes +

Cooking: 10 minutes

Servings: 1

Ingredients

For the chaffles:

- 1 egg
- 1/2 cup Cheddar cheese, shredded

For the sandwich:

- 2 strips bacon
- 1-2 slices tomato
- 2-3 pieces lettuce
- 1 tbspn mayonnaise

Directions

1. Preheat now your waffle maker according to manufacturer Directions.
2. In a tiny mixing bowl, mix egg and shredded cheese. Stir until well combined.

3. Pour one half of the waffle batter into your waffle maker. Cook for 3-4 minutes or until golden brown. Repeat now with the second half of the batter.
4. In a large pan over medium heat, cook the bacon until crispy, turning as needed. Remove now to drain on paper towels.
5. Assemble the sandwich with lettuce, tomato, and mayonnaise. Enjoy!

Nutrition:

Calories: 238, Total Fat: 18g, Saturated Fat: 9g, Unsaturated Fat: 7g, Cholesterol: 143mg, Sodium: 554mg, Carbohydrates: 2g, Fiber: 0g, Sugar: 1g, Protein: 17g

Mini Keto Pizza

Preparation: 5 minutes+

Cooking: 10 minutes

Servings: 2

Ingredients

- 1/2 cup Shredded Mozzarella cheese
- 1 tbspn almond flour
- 1/2 tsp baking powder
- 1 egg
- 1/4 tsp garlic powder
- 1/4 tsp basil
- 2 tbsps low carb pasta sauce
- 2 tbsps mozzarella cheese

Directions

1. While your waffle maker is heating up, in a bowl mix mozzarella cheese, baking powder, garlic, basis, egg and almond flour.
2. Pour 1/2 the mixture into your mini waffle maker.
3. Cook for 3-5 minutes until your pizza waffle is completely cooked. If you check it and the waffle

sticks to your waffle maker let it cook for another minute or two.

4. Next put the remainder of the pizza crust mix into your waffle maker and cook it.

5. Once both pizza crusts are cooked, place them on the baking sheet of your toaster oven.

6. Put 1 tbspn of low carb pasta sauce on top of each pizza crust.

7. Sprinkle 1 tbspn of shredded mozzarella cheese on top of each one.

8. Bake at 350 degrees in the toaster oven for roughly 5 min, just until the cheese is Melt.

Nutrition:

Calories: 195kcal, Carbohydrates: 4g, Protein: 13g, Fat: 14g, Saturated Fat: 6g, Cholesterol: 116mg, Sodium: 301mg, Potassium: 178mg, Fiber: 1g, Sugar: 1g, Vitamin A: 408IU, Calcium: 290mg, Iron: 1mg

Aioli Chicken Chaffle Sandwich

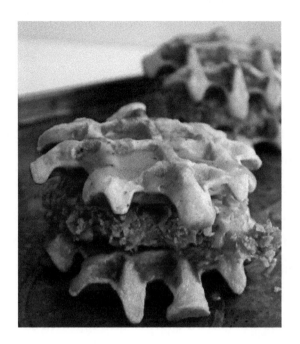

Cooking: 6 Minutes

Servings: 1

Ingredients

- 1/4 cup shredded rotisserie chicken
- 2 Tbsp Kewpie mayo
- 1/2 tsp lemon juice
- 1 grated garlic clove
- 1/4 green onion, chopped

- 1egg
- 1/2 cup shredded mozzarella cheese

Directions

1. Mix lemon juice and mayo in a tiny bowl.
2. Turn on waffle maker to heat and oil it with cooking spray.
3. Beat eggs in a tiny bowl.
4. Place 1/8 cup of cheese on waffle maker, then spread half of the egg mixture over it and top with 1/8 cup of cheese. Close and cook for 3-minutes.
5. Repeat for remaining batter.
6. Place chicken on chaffles and top with sauce. Sprinkle with chopped green onion.

Nutrition:

Carbs: 3 g, Fat: 42 g, Protein: 34 g, Calories: 545

Sage & Coconut Milk Chaffles

Cooking: 24 Minutes

Servings: 6

Ingredients

- 3/4 cup coconut flour, sifted
- 1.1/2 teaspns organic baking powder
- 1/2 teaspn dried ground sage
- 1/8 teaspn garlic powder
- 1/8 teaspn salt
- 1 organic egg
- 1 cup unsweetened coconut milk
- 1/4cup water
- 1/2 tbsps coconut oil, Melt
- 1/2 cup cheddar cheese, shredded

Directions

- Preheat now a waffle iron and then grease it.
- In a bowl, add the flour, baking powder, sage, garlic powder, salt, and mix well.

- Add the egg, coconut milk, water and coconut oil and Mix well until a stiff mixture forms.
- Add the cheese and gently stir to combine.
- Divide the mixture into 6 portions.
- Place 1 portion of the mixture into Preheat waffle iron and cook for about 4 minutes or until golden brown.
- Repeat now with the remaining
- Serve warm.

Nutrition:

Calories: 147, Net Carb: 2.2g, Fat: 13 g, Saturated Fat: 10.7g, Carbohydrates: 2g, Dietary Fiber: 0.7g, Sugar: 1.3g, Protein: 4g

Chaffle Burger

Cooking: 10 Minutes

Servings: 1

Ingredients

For the burger:

- 1/3-pound ground beef
- 1/2 tsp garlic salt
- 2 slices American cheese

For the chaffles:

- 1 large egg
- 1/2 cup shredded mozzarella
- 1/4 tsp garlic salt

For the sauce:

- 2 tsp mayonnaise
- 1 tsp ketchup
- 1 tsp dill pickle relish
- splash vinegar, to taste

For the TOPPINGs:

- 2 Tbsp shredded lettuce
- 3-4 dill pickles

- 2 tsp onion, minced

Directions

1. Heat a skillet over medium-high heat.
2. Divide ground beef into balls and place on the grill, 6 inches apart. cook for 1 minute.
3. Use a tiny plate to flatten beef. Sprinkle with garlic salt.
4. Cook for 2-3, until halfway cooked through. Flip and sprinkle with garlic salt.
5. Cook for 2-3 min, or until cooked completely.
6. Place cheese slice over each patty and stack patties. Set aside on a plate. Cover with foil.
7. Turn on waffle maker to heat and oil it with cooking spray.
8. Whisk egg, cheese, and garlic salt until well combined.
9. Add half of the egg mixture to waffle maker and cook for 2-3 minutes.
10. Set aside and Repeat now with remaining batter.
11. Whisk all sauce ingredientsin a bowl.
12. Top one chaffle with the stacked burger patties, shredded lettuce, pickles, and onions.

13. Spread sauce over the other chaffle and place sauce side down over the sandwich.
14. Eat immediately.

Nutrition:

Calories: 831, Carbs: 8 g, Fat: 5 6 g, Protein: 6 5 g

Best Keto Pizza Chaffle

Preparation: 5 mins

Cooking: 15 mins

Servings: 2

Ingredients

- 1 tsp coconut flour
- 1 egg white
- 1/2 cup mozzarella cheese, shredded
- 1 tsp cream cheese, softened
- 1/4 tsp baking powder
- 1/8 tsp Italian seasoning
- 1/8 tsp garlic powder
- pinch of salt
- 3 tsp low carb marinara sauce
- 1/2 cup mozzarella cheese
- 6 pepperonis cut in half
- 1 tbsp parmesan cheese, shredded
- 1/4 tsp basil seasoning

Directions

1. Preheat now oven to 400 degrees. Turn waffle maker on or plug it in so that it gets hot.

2. A tiny bowl adds coconut flour, egg white, mozzarella cheese, softened cream cheese, baking powder, garlic powder, Italian seasonings, and a pinch of salt.

3. Pour 1/2 of the batter in your waffle maker, close the top, and cook for 3-4 minutes or until chaffle reaches desired doneness.

4. Carefully Remove now chaffle from your waffle maker, then follow the same Directions to make the second chaffle.

5. Top each chaffle with tomato sauce (use 1.1/2 tsp per), pepperoni, mozzarella cheese, and parmesan cheese.

6. Place in the oven on a baking sheet (or straight on the baking rack) on the oven's top shelf for 5-6 minutes. Then turn the oven to broil so that the cheese begins to bubble and brown. Keep a close eye as it can burn quickly. broil for approx 1 min and 30 seconds.

7. Remove now from oven and sprinkle basil on top.

8. Enjoy!

Nutrition:

Calories: 241kcal, Carbohydrates: 4g, Protein: 17g, Fat: 18g, Saturated Fat: 10g , Cholesterol: 49mg, Sodium: 430mg, Potassium: 130mg, Fiber: 1g, Sugar: 1g, Vitamin A: 412IU, Calcium: 339mg, Iron: 1mg

Keto Taco Chaffle with Crispy Taco Shells

Preparation: 5 minutes+

Cooking: 8 mins

Servings: 1

Ingredients

- 1 egg white
- 1/4 cup Monterey jack cheese, shredded (packed tightly)
- 1/4 cup sharp cheddar cheese, shredded (packed tightly)
- 3/4 tsp water
- 1 tsp coconut flour
- 1/4 tsp baking powder
- 1/8 tsp chili powder
- pinch of salt

Directions

1. Plug the Dash Mini Waffle Maker in the wall and grease lightly once it is hot.

2. Combine all of the Ingredients in a bowl and stir to combine.

3. Spoon out 1/2 of the batter on your waffle maker and close lid. Set a timer for 4 minutes and do not lift the lid until the cooking time is complete. If you do, it will look like the taco chaffle shell isn't setting up properly, but it will. You have to let it cook the entire 4 minutes before lifting the lid.

4. Remove now the taco chaffle shell from the waffle iron and set aside. Repeat the same steps above with the rest of the chaffle batter.

5. Turn over a muffin pan and set the taco chaffle shells between the cups to form a taco shell. Allow to set for a few minutes.

6. Remove now and serve with the Very Best Taco Meat or your favorite.

7. Enjoy this delicious keto crispy taco chaffle shell with your favorite TOPPINGs.

Nutrition:

Calories: 258 kcal, Carbohydrates: 4g, Protein: 18g, Fat: 19g, Fiber: 2g, Sugar: 1g

Chaffle Keto Protein Chaffle

Cooking: 8 Minutes

Servings: 1

Ingredients

- 1 egg (beaten)
- 1/2 cup whey protein powder
- A pinch of salt
- 1 tsp baking powder
- 3 tbsp sour cream
- 1/2 tsp vanilla extract

TOPPING:

- 2 tbsp heavy cream
- 1 tbsp granulated swerve

Directions

1. Plug your waffle maker to Preheat now it and spray it with a non-stick cooking spray.
2. In a mixing bowl, whisk together the egg, vanilla and sour cream.

3. In another mixing bowl, combine the protein powder, baking powder and salt.

4. Pour the flour mixture into the egg mixture and Mix well until the Ingredients are well combined and you form a smooth batter.

5. Pour an appropriate amount of the batter into your waffle maker and spread it to the edges to cover all the holes on your waffle maker.

6. Close your waffle maker and cook for about 4 minutes or according to your waffle maker's settings.

7. After the cooking cycle, use a plastic or silicone utensil to Remove now the chaffle from the waffle iron.

8. Repeat step 4 to 6 until you have cooked all the batter into chaffles.

9. For the TOPPING, whisk together the cream and swerve in a mixing bowl until smooth and fluffy.

10. Top the chaffles with the cream and enjoy.

Nutrition:

Fat 25.9g 33%, Carbohydrate 13.1g 5%, Sugars 2.1g, Protein 41.6g

Garlic Mayo Vegan Chaffles

Cooking: 5 minutes

Servings: 2

Ingredients

- 1 tbsp. chia seeds
- 2 ½ tbsps. water
- ¼ cup low carb vegan cheese
- 2 tbsps. coconut flour
- 1 cup low carb vegan cream cheese, softened
- 1 tsp. garlic powder
- pinch of salt
- 2 tbsps. vegan garlic mayo for topping

Directions

1. Preheat now your square waffle maker.
2. In a tiny bowl, mix chia seeds and water, let it stand for 5 minutes.
3. Add all Ingredients to the chia seeds mixture and mix well.
4. Pour vegan chaffle batter in a greased waffle maker

5. Close your waffle maker and cook for about 3-minutesutes.

6. Once chaffles are cooked, Remove now from the maker.

7. Top with garlic mayo and pepper.

8. Enjoy!

Nutrition:

Protein: 32% 42 kcal, Fat: 63% 82 kcal, Carbohydrates: 5% 6 kcal

Best Vegan Keto Chaffle

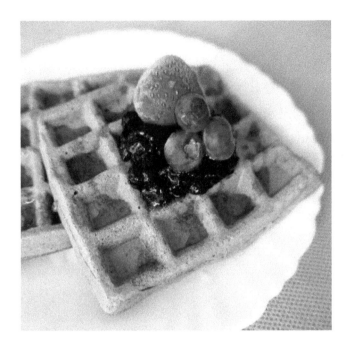

Preparation: 5 minutes

Cooking: 10 minutes

Servings: 2

Ingredients

- ¼ cup of vegan cheese
- 1 tbspn flaxseed meal
- Pinch of salt (as you like)

- 1 tbspn low carb vegan cream cheese, softened
- 2 ½ tbsps of coconut flour

Directions

1. Combine flaxseed meal along with water in a tiny bowl. Let rest for few minutes.
2. Whisk together remaining ingredients. Pour this batter into the center of a Preheat nowed waffle maker and shut with the lid.
3. Cook until golden brown for approx. 3-5 minutes. Serve immediately.

Nutrition:

Fat: 7.3 g, Calories: 114

Cauliflower Chaffles & Tomatoes

Preparation: 5 minutes

Cooking: 10 minutes

Servings: 2

Ingredients

- Cauliflower (.5 cup)
- Black pepper and salt (.25 tsp. each)
- Garlic powder (.25 tsp.)
- Shredded cheddar cheese (.5 cup)
- Egg (1)

The Topping:

- Sliced tomato (1)
- Lettuce leaves (1)
- Steamed - mashed cauliflower (4 oz.)
- Sesame seeds (1 tsp.)

Directions

1. Toss each of the chaffle Ingredients in a blender and thoroughly mix.

2. Warm your waffle maker ahead of cooking time.
3. Drizzle ⅛ teaspn of shredded cheese over the waffle iron grids.
4. Pour in the mixture and add the rest of the cheese.
5. Prepare the chaffles for four to five minutes. Serve with a chaffle, lettuce leaf, and tomato, cauliflower, with a topping of seeds.

Nutrition:

Calories: 198, Net Carbohydrates: 1.73 g, Protein: 12.74 g, Fats: 14.34 g

Broccoli & Cheese Chaffles

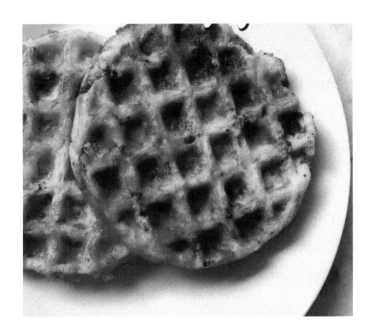

Preparation: 5 minutes

Cooking: 8 minutes

Servings: 2

Ingredients

- ¼ cup broccoli florets
- 1 egg, beaten
- 1 tbspn almond flour
- ¼ teaspn garlic powder

- ½ cup cheddar cheese

Directions

1. Preheat now your waffle maker.
2. Add the broccoli to the food processor.
3. Pulse until chopped.
4. Add to a bowl.
5. Stir in the egg and the rest of the ingredients.
6. Mix well.
7. Pour half of the batter to your waffle maker.
8. Cover and cooking for 4 minutes.
9. Repeat procedure to make the next chaffle.

Nutrition:

Calories 107, Fat 5.4, Fiber 5.6, Carbs 10, Protein 6.8

Scallion - Coconut Chaffles

Preparation: 5 minutes

Cooking: 10 minutes

Servings: 2

Ingredients

- Shredded mozzarella cheese (1 cup)
- Egg (1)
- Cheddar cheese - shredded (1 cup)
- Coconut flour (1.5 tsp.)
- Sliced scallions (2 tbsp.)
- Salt and black pepper (to taste)

Directions

1. Heat a mini waffle maker and spray it using a cooking oil spray.
2. Toss each of the fixings into a bowl and whisk thoroughly.

3. Prepare the batter in two batches, cooking until nicely browned, and serve them right from the cooker.

Nutrition:

Calories: 346, Net Carbohydrates: 7.9 g, Protein: 22.6 g, Fats: 25 grams

Asian Cauliflower Chaffles

Preparation: 9 minutes

Cooking: 28 Minutes

Servings: 2

Ingredients

For the chaffles:

- 1 cup cauliflower rice, steamed
- 1 large egg, beaten
- Salt and freshly ground black pepper to taste
- 1 cup finely grated Parmesan cheese
- 1 tsp sesame seeds
- ¼ cup chopped fresh scallions

For the dipping sauce:

- 3 tbsp coconut aminos
- 1 ½ tbsp plain vinegar
- 1 tsp fresh ginger puree
- 1 tsp fresh garlic paste
- 3 tbsp sesame oil
- 1 tsp fish sauce
- 1 tsp red chili flakes

Directions

1. Preheat now the waffle iron.
2. In a bowl, mix now the cauliflower rice, egg, salt, black pepper, and Parmesan cheese.
3. Open the iron and add a quarter of the mixture. Close and cook until crispy, 7 minutes.
4. Transfer the chaffle to a plate and make 3 more chaffles in the same manner.
5. Meanwhile, make the dipping sauce.
6. In a bowl, mix all the Ingredients for the dipping sauce.
7. Plate the chaffles, garnish with the sesame seeds and scallions and serve with the dipping sauce.

Nutrition:

Calories 427, Total Fat 31.1 g, Saturated Fat 4.2 g, Cholesterol 0 mg, Total Carbs 9 g, Sugar 12.4 g, Fiber 19.8 g, Sodium 86 mg, Potassium 100 mg, Protein 23.5 g

Mushroom and Almond Chaffle

Preparation: 10 minutes

Cooking: 15 minutes

Servings: 4

Ingredients

- 4 eggs
- 2 cups grated Mozzarella cheese
- 1 cup finely chopped zucchini
- 3 tbsps chopped almonds
- 2 teaspns baking powder
- Salt and pepper to taste
- 1 teaspn dried basil
- 1 teaspn chili flakes
- 2 tbsps cooking spray to brush your waffle maker

Directions

1. Preheat now your waffle maker.
2. Add the eggs, grated mozzarella, mushrooms, almonds, baking powder, salt and pepper, dried basil and chili flakes to a bowl.

61

3. Mix with a fork.

4. Brush the heated waffle maker with cooking spray and add a few tbsps of the batter.

5. Close the lid and cooking for about 7 minutes depending on your waffle maker.

6. Serve and enjoy.

Nutrition:

Calories 254, Fat 12, Fiber 3, Carbs 6, Protein 16

Spinach and Artichoke Chaffle

Preparation: 10 minutes

Cooking: 15 minutes

Servings: 4

Ingredients

- 4 eggs
- 2 cups grated provolone cheese
- 1 cup cooked and diced spinach
- ½ cup diced artichoke hearts
- Salt and pepper to taste
- 2 tbsps coconut flour
- 2 teaspns baking powder
- 2 tbsps cooking spray to brush your waffle maker
- ¼ cup of cream cheese for serving

Directions

1. Preheat now your waffle maker.

2. Add the eggs, grated provolone cheese, diced spinach, artichoke hearts, salt and pepper, coconut flour and baking powder to a bowl.
3. Mix with a fork.
4. Brush the heated waffle maker with cooking spray and add a few tbsps of the batter.
5. Close the lid and cooking for about 7 minutes depending on your waffle maker.
6. Serve each chaffle with cream cheese.

Nutrition:

Calories 250, Fat 5, Fiber 7, Carbs 15, Protein 20

Jicama Vegetarian Keto Chaffle

Preparation: 15 minutes

Servings: 2

Ingredients

- Shredded mozzarella cheese (1 cup)
- Lightly beaten eggs (2)
- Onion powder (.25 tsp.) Coconut flour (1.5 tsp.)
- Garlic powder (.25 tsp.)
- Jicama root (1 large - shredded with liquid squeezed out)
- Pepper and salt (to taste)

Directions

1. Preheat now a mini waffle maker.
2. Spray the cooker with a non-stick cooking spray.
3. Shred and add the jicama into a microwave-safe bowl; cook for 5- 8 minutes.
4. Toss in the rest of the fixings to prep the batter.
5. Cook the mixture in two batches and cook until browned (4 min. approx.).

Nutrition:

Calories: 315, Net Carbohydrates: 7.2 g, Protein: 20.1 g, Fats: 23 g

Jicama Loaded Baked Potato Chaffle

Preparation: 10 minutes

Cooking: 15 minutes

Servings: 2

Ingredients

- 1 cup cheese of choice
- 2 eggs, whisked
- 1 large jicama root
- 1/2 medium onion, minced
- Salt and Pepper
- 2 garlic cloves, pressed

Directions

1. Peel jicama and shred in food processor
2. In a large colander, place the shredded jicama, and sprinkle with 1-2 tsp. of salt. Mix well and allow to drain.
3. Squeeze out as much liquid as possible.
4. Microwave for 5-8 minutes
5. Mix all Ingredients

6. Sprinkle a little cheese on waffle iron, then add 1/3 of te mixture, and sprinkle a little more cheese on top of the mixture.
7. Cooking for 5 minutes. Flip and cooking 2 more.
8. Top with a dollop of sour cream, bacon pieces, cheese, and chives.

Nutrition:

Net Carbs: 2.4g; Calories: 321; Total Fat: 21.4g; Saturated Fat: 10.6g; Protein: 27.3g; Carbs: 4.8g; Fiber: 2.4g; Sugar: 1.2g

Lettuce Chaffles Sandwich

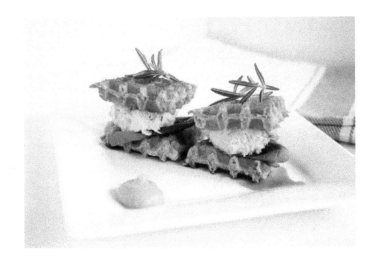

Preparation: 5 minutes

Servings: 2

Ingredients

- Almond flour (1 tbsp.)
- Large egg
- Cheddar cheese - shredded (1 cup)
- Full-fat Greek yogurt (1 tbsp.)
- Baking powder (125 tsp.)
- Shredded Swiss cheese (.25 cup)
- Lettuce leaves (4)

Directions

1. Heat a mini waffle maker and lightly grease it using a cooking oil spray. Whisk the fixings (flour, egg, yogurt, cheese, and baking powder).
2. Dump half of the mixture into the heated cooker for two to three minutes until nicely browned.
3. Use all of the batter and serve them.

Nutrition:

Calories: 180, Net Carbohydrates: 1.81 g, Protein: 10 g, Fats: 14 grams

Vegan Chaffles With Flaxseed

Cooking: 5 minutes

Servings: 2

Ingredients

- 1 tbsp. flaxseed meal
- 2 tbsps. warm water
- 1/4 cup low carb vegan cheese
- 1/4 cup chopped minutest
- pinch of salt
- 2 oz. blueberries chunks

Directions

1. Preheat now waffle maker to medium- high heat and grease with cooking spray.
2. Mix flaxseed meal and warm water and set aside to be thickened.
3. After 5 minutes mix together all Ingredients in flax egg.
4. Pour vegan waffle batter into the center of the waffle iron.

5. Close your waffle maker and let cook for 3-minutes
6. Once cooked, remove now the vegan chaffle from your waffle maker and serve.

Nutrition:

Protein: 32% 42 kcal, Fat: 63% 82 kcal, Carbohydrates: 5% 6 kcal

Crispy Bagel Chaffles

Preparation: 5 minutes

Cooking: 30 Minutes

Servings: 2

Ingredients

- 2 eggs
- ½ cup parmesan cheese
- 1 tsp bagel seasoning
- ½ cup mozzarella cheese
- 2 teaspns almond flour

Directions

1. Turn on waffle maker to heat and oil it with cooking spray.
2. Evenly sprinkle half of cheeses to a skillet and let them Melt now. Then toast for 30 seconds and leave them wait for batter.
3. Whisk eggs, other half of cheeses, almond flour, and bagel seasoning in a tiny bowl.
4. Pour batter into your waffle maker. Cook for minutes.

5. Let cool for 2-3 minutes before serving.

Nutrition:

Calories 117, Fat 2.1g, Carbs 18.2g, Protein 22.7g, Potassium (K) 296mg, Sodium (Na) 81mg, Phosphorous 28 mg

Garlic and Onion Powder Chaffles

Preparation: 5 minutes

Cooking: 5 Minutes

Servings: 2

Ingredients

- 1 organic egg, beaten
- ¼ cup Cheddar cheese, shredded
- 2 tbsps almond flour
- ½ teaspn organic baking powder
- ¼ teaspn garlic powder
- ¼ teaspn onion powder
- Pinch of salt

Directions

1. Preheat now a waffle iron and then grease it.
2. In a bowl, place all the Ingredients and beat until well combined.
3. Place the mixture into Preheat nowed waffle iron and cook for about 5 minutes or until golden brown.

4. Serve warm.

Nutrition:

Calories 249, Protein 12 g, Carbs 30 g, Fat 10 g, Sodium (Na) 32 mg, Potassium (K) 398 mg, Phosphorus 190 mg

Savory Bagel Seasoning Chaffles

Preparation: 10 minutes

Cooking: 5 Minutes

Servings: 4

Ingredients

- 2 tbsps. everything bagel seasoning
- 2 eggs
- 1 cup mozzarella cheese
- 1/2 cup grated parmesan

Directions

1. Preheat now the square waffle maker and grease with cooking spray.
2. Mix eggs, mozzarella cheese and grated cheese in a bowl.
3. Pour half of the batter in your waffle maker.
4. Sprinkle 1 tbsp. of the everything bagel seasoning over batter.
5. Close the lid.
6. Cook chaffles for about 3-4 minutes Utes.

7. Repeat now with the remaining batter.

8. Serve hot and enjoy!

Nutrition:

Calories 64, Fat 3.1, Fiber 3, Carbs 7.1, Protein 2.8

Dried Herbs Chaffle

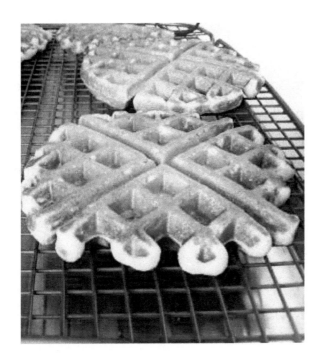

Preparation: 6 minutes

Cooking: 8 Minutes

Servings: 2

Ingredients

- 1 organic egg, beaten
- ½ cup Cheddar cheese, shredded
- 1 tbspn almond flour

- Pinch of dried thyme, crushed
- Pinch of dried rosemary, crushed

Directions

- Preheat now a mini waffle iron and then grease it.
- In a bowl, place all the Ingredients and beat until well combined.
- Place half of the mixture into Preheat waffle iron and cook for about 4 minutes or until golden brown.
- Repeat now with the remaining mixture.
- Serve warm.

Nutrition:

Calories 80, Fat 2.5, Fiber 3.9, Carbs 10.9, Protein 4

Zucchini & Basil Chaffles

Preparation: 6 minutes

Cooking: 10 Minutes

Servings: 2

Ingredients

- 1 organic egg, beaten
- ¼ cup Mozzarella cheese, shredded
- 2 tbsps Parmesan cheese, grated
- ½ of tiny zucchini, grated and squeezed
- ¼ teaspn dried basil, crushed
- Freshly ground black pepper, as required

Directions

1. Preheat now a mini waffle iron and then grease it.
2. In a bowl, place all Ingredients and Mix well until well combined.
3. Place half of the mixture into Preheat nowed waffle iron and cook for about 4-5 minutes or until golden brown.
4. Repeat now with the remaining mixture.

5. Serve warm.

Nutrition:

Calories 43, Fat 3.4, Fiber 1.7, Carbs 3.4, Protein 1.3

Hash Brown Chaffle

Preparation: 6 minutes

Cooking: 10 Minutes

Servings: 2

Ingredients

- 1 large jicama root, peeled and shredded
- ½ medium onion, minced
- 2 garlic cloves, pressed
- 1 cup cheddar shredded cheese
- 2 eggs
- Salt and pepper, to taste

Directions

1. Place jicama in a colander, sprinkle with 2 tsp salt, and let drain.
2. Squeeze out all excess liquid.
3. Microwave jicama for 5-8 minutes.
4. Mix ¾ of cheese and all other Ingredients in a bowl.

5. Sprinkle 1-2 tsp cheese on waffle maker, add 3 Tbsp mixture, and top with 1-2 tsp cheese.
6. Cook for 5-min, or until done.
7. Remove now and repeat for remaining batter.
8. Serve while hot with preferred toppings.

Nutrition:

Calories 81, Fat 4.2, Fiber 6.5, Carbs 11.1, Protein 1.9

Almonds and Flaxseeds Chaffles

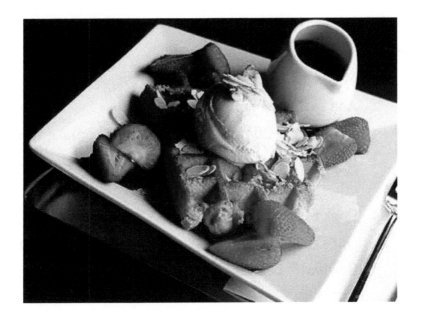

Cooking: 5 minutes

Servings: 2

Ingredients

- 1/4 cup coconut flour
- 1 tsp. stevia
- 1 tbsp. ground flaxseed
- 1/4 tsp baking powder
- 1/2 cup almond milk

- 1/4 tsp vanilla extract
- 1/ cup low carb vegan cheese

Directions

1. Mix flaxseed in warm water and set aside.
2. Add in the remaining Ingredients.
3. Switch on waffle iron and grease with cooking spray.
4. Pour the batter in the waffle machine and close the lid.
5. Cook the chaffles for about 3-4 minutes
6. Once cooked, remove now from the waffle machine.
7. Serve with berries and enjoy!

Nutrition:

Protein: 32% 42 kcal, Fat: 63% kcal, Carbohydrates: 5% 6 kcal

Broccoli Chaffle

Preparation: 10 minutes

Cooking: 15 minutes

Servings: 3 medium chaffles

Ingredients

- 1 cup / 175 grams broccoli florets
- 2 eggs, at room temperature
- 6 tbsps grated parmesan cheese
- 1 cup / 115 grams shredded cheddar cheese

Directions

1. Take a non-stick waffle iron, plug it in, select the medium or medium-high heat setting and let it Preheat now until ready to use; it could also be indicated with an indicator light changing its color.
2. Meanwhile, prepare the batter, and for this, place broccoli florets in a blender and pulse for 1 to 2 minutes until florets resemble rice.
3. Tip the broccoli in a bowl, add remaining Ingredients and then stir with a hand whisk until combined.

4. Use a spoon to pour one-third of the prepared batter into the heated waffle iron in a spiral direction, starting from the edges, then shut the lid and cook for 5 minutes or more until solid and nicely browned; the cooked waffle will look like a cake.

5. When done, transfer chaffles to a plate with a silicone spatula and Repeat now with the remaining batter.

6. Let chaffles stand for some time until crispy and serve straight away.

Garlic Bread Chaffle

Cooking: 15 Minutes

Servings: 2

Ingredients

- 1 tbsp + 1tsp almond flour
- 1 egg
- 14 tsp baking powder
- 1/2 tsp garlic powder
- 1/8 tsp Italian seasoning
- 1 tbsp finely chopped cooked beef liver
- 1/4 tsp garlic salt
- 3 tsp unsalted butter (Melt nowed)
- 1/2 cup shredded mozzarella cheese
- 2 tbsp shredded parmesan cheese

Garnish:

- Chopped green onion

Directions

1. Preheat now the oven to 375°F and line a baking sheet with parchment paper.

2. Plug your waffle maker to Preheat it and spray it with non-stick spray.

3. In a mixing bowl, combine the almond flour, baking powder, Italian seasoning, garlic powder, beef liver and cheese. Add the egg and Mix well until the Ingredients are well combined.

4. Fill your waffle maker with the appropriate amount of the batter and spread the batter to your waffle maker's edges to cover all the holes on the waffle iron.

5. Close your waffle maker's lid and cook for about 3 to 4 minutes or according to waffle maker's settings.

6. Meanwhile, whisk together the garlic salt and melt butter in a bowl.

7. After the cooking cycle, remove now the chaffle from the waffle iron with a plastic or silicone utensil.

8. Repeat step 4, 5 and 7 until you have cooked all the batter into chaffles.

9. Brush the butter mixture over the face of each chaffle.

10. Top the chaffles with parmesan cheese and arrange them into the line baking sheet.

11. Place the sheet in the oven and bake for about 5 minutes or until the cheese melt.

12. Remove now the bread chaffles from the oven and leave them to cool for a few minutes.

13. Serve warm and top with chopped green onions.

Nutrition:

Fat 18g 23%, Carbohydrate 4.59 2%, Sugars 0.9g, Protein 12g

Cinnamon Chaffle Rolls

Preparation: 7 minutes

Cooking: 10 Minutes

Servings: 2

Ingredients

- 1/2 cup mozzarella cheese
- 1 tbsp. almond flour
- 1 egg
- 1 tsp cinnamon
- 1 tsp stevia

Cinnamon Roll Galze:

- 1 tbsp. butter
- 1 tbsp. cream cheese
- 1 tsp. cinnamon
- 1/4 tsp vanilla extract
- 1 tbsp. coconut flour

Directions

1. Switch on a round waffle maker and let it heat up.

2. In a tiny bowl mix together cheese, egg, flour, cinnamon powder, and stevia in a bowl.

3. Spray the round waffle maker with nonstick spray.

4. Pour the batter in a waffle maker and close the lid.

5. Close your waffle maker and cook for about 3-4 minutes Utes.

6. Once chaffles are cooked, Remove now from Maker

7. Mix butter, cream cheese, cinnamon, vanilla and coconut flour in a bowl.

8. Spread this glaze over chaffle and roll up.

9. Serve and enjoy!

Nutrition:

Calories 176, Fat 2.1g, Carbs 27g, Protein 15.1g, Potassium (K) 242mg, Sodium (Na) 72mg, Phosphorous 555.3 mg

Broccoli & Almond Flour Chaffles

Preparation: 6 minutes

Cooking: 8 Minutes

Servings: 2

Ingredients

- 1 organic egg, beaten
- ½ cup Cheddar cheese, shredded
- ¼ cup fresh broccoli, chopped
- 1 tbspn almond flour
- ¼ teaspn garlic powder

Directions

1. Preheat now a mini waffle iron and then grease it.
2. In a bowl, place all Ingredients and mix well until well combined.
3. Place half of the mixture into preheat nowed waffle iron and cook for about 4 minutes or until golden brown.
4. Repeat now with the remaining mixture.
5. Serve warm.

Nutrition:

Calories 221, Protein 17 g, Carbs 31 g, Fat 8 g, Sodium (Na) 235 mg, Potassium (K) 176 mg, Phosphorus 189 mg

Cheddar Jalapeño Chaffle

Preparation: 6 minutes

Cooking: 5 Minutes

Servings: 2

Ingredients

- 2 large eggs
- ½ cup shredded mozzarella
- ¼ cup almond flour
- ½ tsp baking powder
- ¼ cup shredded cheddar cheese
- 2 Tbsp diced jalapeños jarred or canned

For the toppings:

- ½ cooked bacon, chopped
- 2 Tbsp cream cheese
- ¼ jalapeño slices

Directions

1. Turn on waffle maker to heat and oil it with cooking spray.

2. Mix mozzarella, eggs, baking powder, almond flour, and garlic powder in a bowl.

3. Sprinkle 2 Tbsp cheddar cheese in a thin layer on waffle maker, and ½ jalapeño.

4. Spoon half of the egg mixture on top of the cheese and jalapeños.

5. Cook for min, or until done.

6. Repeat for the second chaffle.

7. Top with cream cheese, bacon, and jalapeño slices.

Nutrition:

Calories 221, Protein 13 g, Carbs 1 g, Fat 34 g, Sodium (Na) 80 mg, Potassium (K) 119 mg, Phosphorus 158 mg

Rosemary in Chaffles

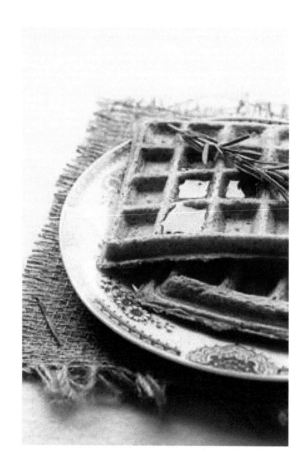

Preparation: 6 minutes

Cooking: 8 Minutes

Servings: 2

Ingredients

- 1 organic egg, beaten
- ½ cup Cheddar cheese, shredded
- 1 tbspn almond flour
- 1 tbspn fresh rosemary, chopped
- Pinch of salt and freshly ground black pepper

Directions

1. Preheat now a mini waffle iron and then grease it.
2. For chaffles: In a bowl, place all Ingredients and Mix well until well combined with a fork.
3. Place half of the mixture into Preheat nowed waffle iron and cook for about 4 minutes or until golden brown.
4. Repeat now with the remaining mixture.
5. Serve warm.

Nutrition:

Calories 221, Protein 12 g, Carbs 29 g, Fat 8 g, Sodium (Na) 398 mg, Potassium (K) 347 mg, Phosphorus 241 mg

Zucchini in Chaffles

Preparation: 10 minutes

Cooking: 18 Minutes

Servings: 2

Ingredients:

- 2 large zucchinis, grated and squeezed
- 2 large organic eggs
- 2/3 cup Cheddar cheese, shredded
- 2 tbsps coconut flour
- ½ teaspn garlic powder
- ½ teaspn red pepper flakes, crushed
- Salt, to taste

Directions

1. Preheat now a waffle iron and then grease it.
2. Place all Ingredients in a bowl and mix until well combined.
3. Place ¼ of the mixture into Preheat nowed waffle iron and cook for about 4-4½ minutes or until golden brown.

4. Repeat now with the remaining mixture.

5. Serve warm.

Nutrition:

Calories 311, Protein 16 g, Carbs 17 g, Fat 15 g, Sodium (Na) 31 mg, Potassium (K) 418 mg, Phosphorus 257 mg

Avocado Croque Madam Chaffle

Cooking: 15 Minutes

Servings: 4

Ingredients

Batter:

- 4 eggs
- 2 cups grated mozzarella cheese
- 1 avocado, mashed
- Salt and pepper to taste
- 6 tbsps almond flour
- 2 teaspns baking powder
- 1 teaspn dried dill

Other:

- 2 tbsps cooking spray to brush your waffle maker
- 4 fried eggs
- 2 tbsps freshly chopped basil

Directions

1. Preheat now your waffle maker.

2. Add the eggs, grated mozzarella, avocado, salt and pepper, almond flour, baking powder and dried dill to a bowl.
3. Mix with a fork.
4. Brush the heated waffle maker with cooking spray and add a few tbsps of the batter.
5. Close the lid and cook for about 7 minutes depending on your waffle maker.
6. Serve each chaffle with a fried egg and freshly chopped basil on top.

Nutrition:

Calories 393, fat 32.1 g, carbs 9.2 g, sugar 1.3 g, Protein 18.8 g, sodium 245 mg

Fruity Vegan Chaffles

Cooking: 5 minutes

Servings: 2

Ingredients

- 1 tbsp. chia seeds
- 2 tbsps. warm water
- ¼ cup low carb vegan cheese
- 2 tbsps. strawberry puree
- 2 tbsps. Greek yogurt
- pinch of salt

Directions

1. Preheat now the waffle maker to medium-high heat.
2. In a tiny bowl, mix chia seeds and water and let it stand for few minutes to be thickened.
3. Mix now the rest of the Ingredients in chia seed egg and mix well.
4. Spray waffle machine with cooking spray.
5. Pour vegan waffle batter into the center of the waffle iron.

6. Close your waffle maker and cook chaffles for about 3-5 minutes.
7. Once cooked, remove now from the maker and serve with berries on top.

Nutrition:

Protein: 32% 42 kcal, Fat: 63% kcal, Carbohydrates: 5% 6 kcal

Vegan Chocolate Chaffles

Cooking: 5minutes

Servings: 2

Ingredients

- 1/2 cup coconut flour
- 3 tbsps. cocoa powder
- 2 tbsps. whole psyllium husk
- 1/2 teaspn baking powder
- pinch of salt
- 1/2 cup vegan cheese, softened
- 1/4 cup coconut milk

Directions

- Prepare your waffle iron according to the manufacturer's Directions.
- Mix coconut flour, cocoa powder, baking powder, salt and husk in a bowl and set aside.
- Add melt cheese and milk and mix well. Let it stand for a few minutes before cooking.

- Pour batter in waffle machine and cook for about 3-minutes.
- Once chaffles are cooked, carefully remove now them from the waffle machine.
- Serve with vegan ice cream and enjoy!

Nutrition:

Protein: 32% 42 kcal, Fat: 63% 82 kcal, Carbohydrates: 5% 6 kcal

Apple Cinnamon Chaffles

Preparation: 6 minutes

Cooking: 20 Minutes

Servings: 2

Ingredients

- 3 eggs, lightly beaten
- 1 cup mozzarella cheese, shredded
- ¼ cup apple, chopped
- ½ tsp monk fruit sweetener
- 1 ½ tsp cinnamon
- ¼ tsp baking powder, gluten-free
- 2 tbsp coconut flour

Directions

- Preheat now your waffle maker.
- Add remaining Ingredients and stir until well combined.
- Spray waffle maker with cooking spray.
- Pour 1/3 of batter in the hot waffle maker and cook for minutes or until golden brown. Repeat now with the remaining batter.

- Serve and enjoy.

Nutrition:

Calories 227, Fat 18.6, Fiber 4.5, Carbs 9.5, Protein 9.9

Blueberry Chaffles

Preparation: 8 minutes

Cooking: 15 Minutes

Servings: 2

Ingredients

- 2 eggs
- 1/2 cup blueberries
- 1/2 tsp baking powder
- 1/2 tsp vanilla
- 2 tsp Swerve
- 3 tbsp almond flour
- 1 cup mozzarella cheese, shredded

Directions

1. Preheat now your waffle maker.
2. In a bowl, mix eggs, vanilla, Swerve, almond flour, and cheese.
3. Add blueberries and stir well.
4. Spray waffle maker with cooking spray.

5. Pour 1/4 batter in the hot waffle maker and cook for 8 minutes or until golden brown. Repeat now with the remaining batter.
6. Serve and enjoy.

Nutrition:

Calories 96, Fat 6.1g, Carbohydrates 5g, Sugar 2.2g, Protein 6.1g, Cholesterol 86 mg

9 781802 699180